# Balance 2.0

# Also by Amanda Sterczyk

*Your Job Is Killing You:*
*A User's Guide to Sneaking Exercise into Your Work Day*

*Balance and Your Body:*
*How Exercise Can Help You Avoid a Fall*

*Move More, Your Life Depends On It:*
*Practical Tips to Add More Movement to Your Day*

*I Can See Your Underwear:*
*My Journey Through the Fitness World*

*For more information,*
*please visit amandasterczyk.com.*

# Balance 2.0

## Preventing Falls
## with Exercise

Amanda Sterczyk

Foreword by Suzanne Reid

The information in this book should not be used for diagnosis or treatment, or as a substitute for professional medical care. Before beginning any exercise program, consult your physician.

Sterczyk, Amanda, author
  Balance 2.0: Preventing Falls with Exercise.


Includes bibliographical references.
Issued in print and electronic formats.

ISBN 9798613201051

  1. Aging. 2. Fall Prevention 3. Physical Fitness
4. Healthy Aging 5. Balance Training


Editor: Kaarina Stiff
Cover: Dianna Little, cover image: iStock Photo
Exercise Illustrations: Emily Sterczyk
Layout: Matthew Bin
Author photo: Allison Mundle
Published by Kindle Direct Publishing

May you live a long and healthy life,

free from slips, trips, and broken hips.

And falls.



Move more, feel better.

# CONTENTS

# FOREWORD

Working as a Registered Physiotherapist for the past 31 years, it has been my good fortune to follow clients over the course of multiple decades and through a variety of important life events, not to mention the bevy of musculo-skeletal injuries to which we, as humans, are prone.

Through this lens, I have seen many of my clients "evolve" from physically active mid-lifers who, over time and often in response to a variety of factors (such as injury, illness, aging, social isolation, etc.), gradually adopt a more sedentary lifestyle—moving less, experiencing more joint stiffness, losing balance skills, and suffering from muscular weakness and diminished kinesthetic and proprioceptive awareness (meaning knowledge of how their joints are moving and where they are in space).

Over time, and as a result of multiple factors (as Amanda has beautifully described in this book), our bal-ance reactions diminish and, ultimately, we become far more vulnerable to falls, fractures and the sequelae related to these injuries, such as chronic pain, reduced mobility, disability and an increasing degree of dependence.

According to the Public Health Agency of Canada, ap-proximately one-quarter of seniors suffer a fall every year. They have further reported that, while hip fractures (and resulting hospitalizations) are the most common result of falls in seniors, broken bones or fractures occur in the vast majority of falls.[1] We also know that 28 per cent of women and 37 per cent of men who suffer a hip fracture will die within one year.[2] These statistics are indeed both cause for serious concern and a call to action.

Amanda's book, *Balance 2.0*, is a remedy for our fear, a tool for change, and a light amongst all those grim statistics because in it, she outlines a prescription for a guided therapeutic exercise program that will safely increase your muscle strength, improve your posture, assist with activities of daily living (such as reaching, squatting, climbing stairs, turning, walking, etc.) and ultimately decrease our risk of falling.

One section of the book that really stood out for me as a clinician was the personal journey of Amanda working with her father, Alex, who experienced a very familiar story of illness, hospitalizations and ensuing weakness, frailty, postural changes and loss of balance—all putting him at increased risk of falling. What I found most poignant about this story is how relevant it is to each and every one of us, whether we are caring for aging parents or are experiencing these changes first-hand. As Amanda

1. Public Health Agency of Canada, Seniors' Falls in Canada: Second Report (Ottawa: Government of Canada, 2014), https://www.canada.ca/en/public-health/services/health-promotion/aging-seniors/publications/publications-general-public/seniors-falls-canada-second-report.html.

2. Osteoporosis Canada (website) Osteoporosis Fast Facts, access January 11, 2020, osteoporosis.ca/about-the-disease/fast-facts.

recounts their interactions so skillfully and compassionately, we are witness to the profound changes that can accompany simple, basic exercises that can easily be done in your own home and with no need for specialized equipment. Alex slowly and surely regained his strength, improved his posture. The positive effects then snowballed from there: His balance improved, risk of falls decreased, confidence for movement grew and he was increasingly motivated to continue his daily exercise. This, in turn, will have far-reaching effects on his bone health, cardiovascular health, brain health, sleep, mood, optimal weight…the list is endless.

I highly recommend this book! Let Amanda help you move more, stay strong and balanced, stand proud, maintain independence and THRIVE.

Suzanne Reid
Registered Physiotherapist & Co-Founder
Killens Reid Physiotherapy Clinic, Ottawa, Canada

# INTRODUCTION

*Old age isn't so bad when you consider the alternative.*

*- Maurice Chevalier, French singer (1888-1972)*

My sister died young when we were both in our twenties. As tragic as it was for her, it forced me to rewrite my plans for my future self—and fast. You see, we had grown up with two maternal great aunts in our sphere. They were widowed and childless, living near each other, but not so close as to be in each other's hair. They lived in the same complex but in separate apartment buildings. My sister and I had always seen ourselves following this path, like a modern-day Auntie Addie and Auntie Liz—connected yet independent in our old age.

I always saw myself as Auntie Addie, the stronger one who continued using the complex's indoor pool into her eighties. As a child, I was a fish, opting for swimming whenever possible. Though, these days, my preferred go-to exercise is walking, I like to get my body moving every day. For me, there's nothing like a brisk walk to oil creaky joints and clear my mind. But you get my point: The idea of moving and staying physically active into my later years felt completely natural, even to my childlike sensibilities.

As we age, we tend to slow down. Our muscles shrink, our vision blurs, and our reaction time diminishes. Together, all of these factors lead to an increased risk of falling. But it doesn't need to be that way. This book, along with *Balance and Your Body: How Exercise Can Help You*

*Avoid a Fall,* provides a plan to keep your muscles strong and your confidence high. We all need bodies that will support our weight as we move through life. Our confidence in our ability to maintain an upright position—i.e., to *not* fall—is just as important.

My hope with my balance books is to rebuild your confidence *and* your muscles, so that you can enjoy your golden years. You deserve as much, and I want to help you get there.

If you read *Balance and Your Body* and followed along with the exercises in that book, I'll tell you now: The exercises in this book are completely different. You will see some repetition in the statistics and the information about the impact of falls on seniors, but those things are worth reading again. Why? These facts are crucial to understanding what could become an epidemic of falls in the older adult population. However, there's lots of fresh material here for you to absorb. In my first *Balance* book, the exercises addressed your balance system, strength, posture, and joint mobility. What's new in this book is the exercises. This set focuses specifically on lower limb strength to improve walking, upper body strength to reinforce good posture, and various arm reaches to improve ease of movement during your day-to-day life.

This book, just like the first *Balance* book, includes a series of functional exercises—more simple, basic, and easy movements that can be done in your home, without the need for special equipment. The exercise instructions also include guidance on how to visualize the movement, to further build linkages between your brain and body.

I wanted to keep the theory in this follow-up book shorter so you can get right to exercising for fall prevention. On that note, let's get to it.

# PART ONE
# THE PROBLEM: FALLING

*Growing old is no more than a bad habit*
*which a busy man has no time to form.*
*- André Maurois, French writer (1885-1967)*

## What's the Problem with Falling?

Falls are no fun, especially as you age. They can lead to injuries such as broken bones, cuts, and concussions. The older you are, the more likely you are to fall. In Canada, falls are the leading cause of injury among older Canadians: 20 to 30 per cent of seniors experience one or more falls each year. In fact, falls are the cause of 85 percent of seniors' injury-related hospitalizations. You may also be surprised to learn that falls are the cause of 95 percent of all hip fractures, and fully half of all falls causing hospitalization happen at home.[1]

In the United States, data reported by the National Council on Aging show that one-quarter of Americans

---

1. Public Health Agency of Canada, You CAN Prevent Falls! (Ottawa: Government of Canada, 2005, Revised 2015), https://www.canada.ca /en/public-health/services/health-promotion/aging-seniors/publications/ publications-general-public/you-prevent-falls.html. Reprinted with permission from the Minister of Health, 2019.

over the age of 65 will fall each year. Falls are also the prevailing reason for hospital admissions among the elderly. An emergency room in the United States treats a senior fall victim every 11 seconds. And, if you're an older adult, you're more likely to die from a fall than any other cause.[2] In the past, research attributed the risk of falls exclusively to aging. That is to say, the likelihood of a fall was simply connected to the year we were born. In truth, it's more like aging *and* lack of physical activity are working together to increase the likelihood that we will fall. As we age, we are typically less active. Our bodies get weaker, our bones get more brittle, and that is why we're more likely to fall. And when we do suffer a fall later in life, we're also more likely to be injured.

That's why I wrote my first book about fall prevention, *Balance and Your Body: How Exercise Can Help You Avoid a Fall*, and that's why you're now reading my second book on the topic. I don't want you to fall. In my role as a personal trainer and group fitness instructor specializing in seniors' fitness, I gained a lot of experience working with older adults just like you. But as you'll see later on, I recently began working one-on-one with my most important client. He, like you, wants to maintain his independence and he realized that preventing a nasty tumble was key to his goal. I hope you'll feel the same way, and follow the exercises to maintain good health and independence.

---

2. National Council on Aging (website), Falls Prevention Facts, accessed March 22, 2019, https://www.ncoa.org/news/resources-for-reporters/get-the-facts/falls-prevention-facts/.

In the next few sections, I'll explain the key factors in balance and fall prevention. Not to worry, though, as there won't be a test of your knowledge at the end! I'm simply sharing the information to help you understand the complexity of our balance system and the importance of our muscles.

## What's Involved in Balance?

*Our body is a machine for living.*
*It is organized for that, it is its nature.*
*- Leo Tolstoy, Russian writer (1828-1910)*

While this isn't strictly a new chapter, I love this quote and I believe it's highly relevant to a discussion about balance. What is balance, anyway? Basically, balance means your weight is distributed in such a way that you can maintain an upright posture. But that doesn't mean you're a stiff, two-dimensional robot that is always in the same upright position. We move our bodies in unique, dynamic ways as we move through life. And the goal—well, my goal, and I hope yours too—is to keep ourselves from falling as we move through life.

So what's involved in balance? I'm glad you asked, because it's fascinating how seemingly disparate systems in our body work together to maintain balance. Our balance system is complex and relies on sensory input from three distinct systems: visual, vestibular, and proprioceptive (also known as somatosensory). All of this is just a fancy way of describing how our bodies process information. Let me break them down.

Visual system: As you might guess, this is about our eyes, which provide visual input to our brains as we move through life.

Vestibular system: This is the medical term for the inner ear, which processes sensory information about motion, equilibrium, and spatial orientation. Close your eyes and slowly move your head side to side. Your vestibular system is now sending crucial input to your brain. As we age, our side-to-side head movements become less frequent, which negatively impacts our vestibular system. In other words, it doesn't work if we don't use it. "Use it or lose it" doesn't just apply to our muscles—it applies to every single part of our bodies.

Proprioception or somatosensory: This is our brain's ability to sense our body's position in space. That's why we can walk through our house in the dark without falling down, unless of course, we bang into an unseen (because it's dark) object or trip over the cat. The nerves in our body send signals to our brain that allow us to maintain an upright position, and we have just as many sensors (i.e., nerve endings) in the bottom of our feet as we do in our entire spinal column.

So what does it mean to be balanced? It's when you can maintain your centre of gravity over your base of support, whether you are standing or moving.[3] Good balance

3. Jiejiao Zheng et al., "Strategic targeted exercise for preventing falls in elderly people," *Journal of International Medical Research* 41, no. 2 (2013):

relies on strength. You need strong muscles and bones to keep you upright, whether you're moving around or just standing still. And that's a problem as we age, because we are prone to sarcopenia, which I'll explain next.

## Sarco-what?

No one sets out to get weak. It just happens. And the problem is that our own bodies sometimes work against us. As we celebrate more birthdays, sarcopenia takes more of our strength. If you're thinking "sarco-what?!", let me elaborate.

Sarcopenia is age-related muscle loss that contributes to frailty, loss of strength, and inevitably, falls.[4] This decline begins in our 40s and follows a fairly straight pattern—each year, we lose more muscle. Have you noticed your legs getting skinnier, more spindly, every year? That's what sarcopenia looks like. By the time you're in your seventies, you've lost half the mass in your muscles.

One of the best ways to fight this loss of muscle tissue is with resistance or strength training.[5] Lower limb strength means your legs are able to carry you as you stand and walk. Those same legs need to be strong enough to step up to climb stairs, balance you as you shift weight from one foot to the other when you walk, and when you

---

418-426, https://journals.sagepub.com/doi/pdf/10.1177/0300060513477297.

4. Jeremy Walston, "Sarcopenia in Older Adults," *Curr Opin Rheumatol*, 26, no. 6 (November 2012): 623-627, 10.1097/BOR.0b013e328358d59b.

5. Walston, "Sarcopenia," 2012.

move from sitting to standing. Your upper body also needs to be strong in order to hold you upright and resist momentum and gravity, which would topple you over if you stoop too far forward. These upper body muscles also help you maintain an upright posture as you reach, twist, or turn during your everyday activities.

The targeted exercises included in this book will help you strengthen both your lower limbs and upper body muscles, which goes a long way to fighting back against sarcopenia.

## When Is It Time for Medical Assistance?

As a fitness professional, I often have clients asking for advice that goes beyond my knowledge base. As my friend, athletic trainer Cassandra McCoy, always says, "When in doubt, refer out." Meaning, medical advice is beyond my scope of practice. In these cases, I recommend that the client speaks with their doctor, physical or athletic therapist, or other health professional.

Once they have a diagnosis and treatment plan, I'm happy to work with them on their exercises. I recommend the same for you. If you try the exercises in this book and you struggle, or if you get dizzy and the feeling won't go away, please STOP and consult a health professional.

I asked another friend and athletic therapist, Mélanie Fiala, to weigh in on the topic. Mel works with men, women and children of all ages, amateur and professional athletes, as well as what she likes to call "real people": members of the general public. As Mélanie well knows, there are age-related deficiencies in our balance system that can be corrected with exercises such as the ones you'll find later in this book. For the occasions when exercise is not enough, it's time to ask for help. So I asked Mel to help you understand when it's time to pick up the phone and book an appointment with a medical professional. The information below is taken from our interview.[6]

**Q:** While it is normal for people to experience dizziness occasionally, sometimes it is cause for concern, particularly when starting a new routine.When does general dizziness need to be addressed by a medical professional?

**A:** "Even if someone has spoken to their doctor about dizziness before, they should follow-up with a medical professional if:

- the dizziness is changing—for example, if it becomes more frequent, lasts longer, or feels different,
- it is accompanied by other symptoms,
- it's not related to any preexisting or known medical conditions, such as low or high blood pressure, vertigo, or hypoglycemia (low blood sugar),
- it's related to a pre-existing or known medical condition and it has changed,
- they have recently suffered a head injury or a fall (the dizziness could be related even if they didn't hit their head),

---

6. Online interview conducted with Mélanie Fiala, CAT (C), via email December 2019.

- it is accompanied by any other neurological symptoms, such as numbness, tingling, or double vision, or

- they experience a fall from dizziness.

Bottom line, if someone is unsure and it's not something they have experienced before, it is never a bad idea to have these signs and symptoms checked by a medical professional."

**Q:** If a senior experiences dizziness or weakness when following a home exercise plan, how would you advise them to proceed?

**A:** "If this occurs often, is changing or getting worse, they should talk to their health care professional about it. Experiencing dizziness while working out can be dangerous. I always remind people: Check your breathing! Are you holding your breath? Are you breathing at a different pace than usual? This can cause unnecessary and sudden elevation in blood pressure which can be related to dizziness. They should pay attention to the repetitions they are doing. If they're overdoing it, they could experience dizziness."

**Q:** Our balance system diminishes as we age. In your experience, what helps most to counter the effects of aging?

**A:** "I like to tell people, 'Move or you'll rust!' The more they use their brain and body in a way that requires balance, the more their body will adapt and stay balanced."

Mel has provided us with valuable information that I hope you'll keep in mind as you tackle the exercises in this book.

## Do You Have Young Legs?

"Who's got young legs?!"

That's how my grandmother used to call out to us kids when she needed one of us to fetch something from the basement. One of the grandchildren would run down and then back up the stairs with whatever she needed. I can't speak for my siblings, but their basement scared the heck out of me. I was convinced some type of gremlin dwelt there, so my young legs moved me back up those stairs as quickly as possible.

However, we were only there on the weekends to help with our young legs. Five days a week, my grandmother had to rely on her own young legs to store food in the freezer, fetch other food from the cold storage, not to mention loads of laundry up and down and up and down. You get the idea. She went up and down the stairs quite a bit.

She didn't have a fancy stair-climber, like the ones you see at the gyms these days. She just had a two-storey house with a basement, no dishwasher, no garage door opener, no television remote, no cordless phone, and an incredibly heavy vacuum cleaner to boot. Having no modern conveniences meant that she had young legs by the very nature of her daily life.

So if your memory is waning and you often forget something in another part of your home, thank your rusty brain for helping your young legs. And use it as an excuse to get up and move more. After all, that's what your body was designed to do.

## Is Multi-tasking the Answer?

Can you walk and chew gum? This question is only slightly frivolous, because walking is the ultimate multi-tasking activity. Think about it: You constantly shift your weight from one foot to the other and back again. To successfully accomplish this dynamic balance work, your muscles need to be strong enough to continuously lift your feet and clear the ground safely. Your bones and the muscles in your torso must be strong enough to maintain an upright posture. And your balance is being continuously challenged as you shift your centre of gravity and base of support (more on those concepts later). Walking is multi-tasking at its best, if you ask me.

But not all multi-tasking is beneficial or even safe. Take balance challenges, for example. I've seen a number of people advocate for balancing when you're doing daily tasks, such as balancing on one foot while you're brushing your teeth. Their reasoning goes something like this: You're standing in your bathroom, with a counter nearby for support, for at least two minutes—if you're following your dentist's recommendation, that is—otherwise, maybe your time in the bathroom is more like one minute long. In any case, these well-meaning souls recommend you stand on one foot *while* you're brushing your teeth.

Think about that for a moment: You're already balance-challenged, you have something in your mouth, and you're going to try to hold that position without falling over. What would your mother say? That's right, she would tell you you're being foolhardy and careless, hopping around on one foot with something long and pointy in your mouth.

And she's not wrong, either. I know someone who, as a teenager, was doing just that—hopping around with a pencil in their mouth. I'll bet you can guess what happened. They ended up in the hospital emergency department with a pencil lodged in the back of their throat. Fortunately, it didn't cause permanent damage. Now, before you try to discount the risk with a toothbrush by arguing that it's much bigger than a pencil, I'm going to stop you right there. Do you really want to take that chance? Are you feeling lucky? I suggest we dispense with the overly complicated multi-tasking and instead focus on exercises that can be completed safely!

## What Happened in the Workshops?

When I wrote my first exercise book, *Balance and Your Body: How Exercise Can Help You Avoid a Fall*, the content came out of a workshop on seniors' fall prevention that I was asked to give at a local community health centre. While researching and creating the slides, I quickly realized that the content would translate well into an exercise guide for home use.

So I got to writing and asked my mother-in-law to be my exercise guinea pig as I fine-tuned the exercise instructions. It worked well and I've received great feedback from men and women who have benefited from the book, as well as younger adults who have used it to help their aging loved ones remain strong and prevent falls.

After *Balance and Your Body* was released, I was hired by our local library to deliver more fall prevention classes based on the exercises in that book. They are basic, easy-to-follow sequences that don't require special equipment. These workshops were well received by participants. The feedback collected at the end of the sessions included things like:

- "Please bring Amanda back for more workshops."
- "These exercises are so important and helpful."
- "We want more easy-to-follow exercises—please write another book!"

You get the idea: The sessions were a success, and I sold out of the books I had brought with me. The seed was planted to create a second book of balance exercises. It wasn't until my father landed in the hospital a few months later that this second book finally came to fruition. I'll get into his story in the next section.

The reason I mention the workshops is this: What is written in the exercise section is the same information I use to teach these exercises to seniors in person. This includes step-by-step instructions, modifications to make the sequences easier or harder, and visual cues to help you with proper positioning. But don't take my word for it—arrange your own mini workshop with friends or loved ones to practice the exercises. You can take turns reading the instructions and appraising each other's execution. Heck, if you want to get fancy, grab your smartphone and record short videos of each other. Watch the feedback together to help you improve. That's how the professional athletes do it.

The other feedback I received from workshop participants and readers of my first balance book is this: Give us more! Seniors who are concerned about falling know it's a problem that could soon become an epidemic. They told me they don't need lots of information on the problem with falling because they know that firsthand already. Rather, they asked me for more exercises they could do at home, more ways they could strengthen their bodies without needing any special equipment or fancy workout clothing. At one of the workshops, I showed up in fancy dress pants and a sweater, to demonstrate that you really could do the exercises anytime, anywhere, dressed in regular clothing. So while this book is a little light on the research around falling, my first book has all the data to cover those bases. Here, we're going to focus on how to not fall. And I'll share with you how I helped my father reduce his fall risk with a targeted exercise plan, a plan similar to the one in this book.

# PART TWO
# THE SOLUTION: NOT FALLING

*It is better to be seventy years young*
*than forty years old!*
*- Oliver Wendell Holmes, American poet (1809-1894)*

## Can I Tell You About My Father?

My father, Alex, had a tough go of it over a one-year period with four multi-day hospital visits. Fortunately, none of these stopovers were the result of a fall. But he had still lost substance: He lost weight, lost height, lost strength, lost muscle mass. My mother and I were concerned that the last two stays, especially, put him at high risk for a fall. It was, after all, late autumn with an early snow cover and all that that entails, such as:

- Heavier coats that weigh you down and tire you out,
- Clunky boots that require you to lift your foot that much higher to clear sidewalks, snowbanks, and the edge of the car, and
- Slippery sidewalks and driveways that unsteady you and sap your confidence in your ability to stay upright.

Up until his fourth visit, I was offering suggestions about ways he could regain strength and muscle, but from a distance. I didn't want to insert myself if he wasn't prepared to have me work with him. Maybe the same thing has happened in your family, either as a parent or adult child. But after his fourth visit, I decided it was time to intervene. I was concerned for his safety, and I was qualified to help him. It's what I've done with my senior clients, so now I was taking on my most important client ever.

My father agreed to have me come visit twice the following week, on a consecutive Tuesday and Wednesday. As I would with any client, I drew up a training plan before our first visit. He wanted to work on core strength as well as leg strength, and he told me that he had to physically lift his leg in and out of the car with his hands. I agreed that these were fitting goals and we got to work.

I explained to my father that we would limit his exercise time to 30 minutes at each visit. On the first day, he learned and practiced six exercises, followed by a 10-minute ride on his stationary bike. Since the bike is in his bedroom, it's an immediate reminder for him to move more, and I recommended that he try to use the bike for 10 minutes every day, especially on the days when I wasn't coming over.

I asked my father if he had done any of the exercises from my first book, *Balance and Your Body*. He admitted that he hadn't tried them in some time. I pulled his copy off the nightstand and flipped to the section on active sitting, explaining how important it was to not slouch in a chair. He nodded as I spoke, and disclosed that he had been working on both his seated and standing posture as a way to alleviate his low back pain. And it was working, he told me. Another fitness win, in my opinion!

As I was leaving at the end of our first session, my dad was getting ready to climb on his bike. I bid him adieu, promising to return at the same time tomorrow.

## Day Two: Did He Get Stronger?

The next day, I already witnessed an improvement in my father. I've written before about how people who have been previously sedentary have the most to gain from adding even a small amount of exercise to their life. And here I was, observing it first-hand with my most important client. My dad was motivated and we covered twice as many exercises as we had the day before. That's not to say we rushed through our 30-minute session. On the contrary, slow and steady was our mantra.

The day before, I had guided him through exercises on his back—lying on his bed, not the floor—and seated in a chair. Today, though, I wanted him to complete a series of standing exercises, so two-thirds of the exercises were of the standing variety. After a water break, we opted to have him sit down to finish the workout.

I was excited to see that he was keen to keep going. He was stronger and more energized too, observations that I shared with him. My father noted that the exercises I was teaching him were tough, but he could feel that they were already helping him.

We talked about the importance of avoiding a fall, and how people his age risk a second fall within 12 months of their first fall. Every health care professional he had seen in the past year asked him if he had fallen. That's not surprising, since seniors are more likely to fall than their younger counterparts, and the risk of falling increases every year. He told me what he tells these practitioners:

"My daughter has made me very aware of fall prevention. So I take care to move cautiously, working to keep control of my body."

You know how parents are often proud of their kids? This was a case where I was so proud of my dad! He wasn't just listening to my advice—he was acting on it too!

## Day Three: Was He Walking Better?

Our third session happened three days later, on a Saturday afternoon. We focused on standing-only exercises. Once again, my dad impressed me with his commitment to good form and execution of the moves. As we finished our 30 minutes, he stood up to walk to the washroom. I noticed right away that he was standing taller and moving more easily than when we had started.

I said, "You're walking better," to which he replied, "I feel like I have better balance."

Yes, he did have better balance.

## What Happened in Week Two?

It was week two, our fourth day of working together. My mother greeted me at the door, saying, "Thank you for doing this."

She was feeling positive about his progress, and it showed. The stress and uncertainty of a loved one potentially falling and injuring themselves weighs on many people's minds. I can tell you that even small strength gains and progress were putting everyone's minds at ease.

My mother told me that my father had already completed his 10 minutes on the bicycle. He definitely had more energy when we finally started the exercises, after only one week with three 30-minute sessions.

We were able to double the number of repetitions he completed on my last visit. Think about that for a moment: He went from doing 10 heel raises to doing 20 heel raises. He told me that he could feel his muscles working.

Another incredible thing happened as we completed the exercise sequences. Every time I was about to correct his form, he would beat me to it. My dad would pause and comment that he felt like he was leaning forward, or slouched, or uneven in his shoulders, and then he would correct his positioning before continuing the exercise.

Call it body awareness, self-awareness, whatever you'd like. I'll tell you the official terminology: It's proprioception and it means you are aware of your body's position and how you're moving it. That's an important concept to grasp and an even more important concept to learn, because it directly impacts your balance and your ability to avoid a fall. Hurray!

I asked my father if he was noticing any changes since we had started, only one week earlier. His told me:

"I'm using my walker less, my back is hurting less, and I feel stronger."

Double hurray!

Later that day, my father had a medical appointment, and the staff at the clinic noticed how improved he was. They said things like,

"Oh my, he is walking so much better!" and

"He looks straighter."

I went over twice more during our second week of targeted exercises—on a Friday and Sunday. And do you know what had happened on the intervening day? My father completed exercises on his own, even marking them down on his training tracking log. He was beginning to feel more confident and he was willing to work out solo. In the back of this book, you will find a training log that you can use to track the first two weeks of your progress with these exercises. I hope this visual nudge will encourage you to keep going. You can do it!

## What About Week Three?

On more than one occasion, our sessions together lasted less than 30 minutes. Although I would like my father to exercise for 30 minutes a day for at least three days a week, that's only a goal, not a hard and fast rule. If he seems like he's struggling to complete the exercises safely, we stop, take a rest, and reassess. Sometimes, we move on to another exercise, other times, we call it a day. It's sound advice that I hope you will also heed.

It can be foolhardy to "power through" if you're not feeling 100 per cent. You risk injuring yourself and even falling, which is completely counterproductive in a fall prevention program! One day, my father was completing the heel-toe walk and he stumbled. He was having more difficulty with the exercise than he had had just a few days prior. I immediately called for a break and helped him to sit down, suggesting that we switch to the lying exercises, to which he agreed. So, listen to your body and the cues it is telling you.

In his first week of targeted exercises, he experienced a tremendous gain in strength and confidence. Others around him were noticing and commenting on his stronger, more upright form. As a result, we were both overly ambitious about his abilities that day. I pointed out that, at his age, fitness progress can and should be tracked in two ways: peaks and steps.

A peak is when you improve—a lot—from your pre-exercise state. You notice it, others notice it, and it motivates you to keep going. When you have been previously sedentary, your first peak will happen quite quickly. It's a great self-confidence boost too.

On a step, you may feel like you've hit a plateau, but that's better than the alternative, which is a downward slide. If you've been prone to significant age-related muscle mass and bone density loss, you need to be realistic about your progress. By that I mean, you may feel like you're stuck on a step, not improving. But I'm here to tell you that maintaining this new level—staying on this step—is, in fact, progress. I hope that my message will compel you to keep going with the exercises.

In my father's case, I regretted that I pushed him that day and made a commitment to both of us to ease off at our next session. He thanked me for my time and we bid adieu until the next session, three days hence.

I hope you will also practice patience with yourself as you learn these exercises. Some days, you may only want to complete as few as one or two, while other days, you may want to do a full thirty-minute session. Either way, every minute of movement counts and gets you stronger and more confident. That's the goal of this book—to keep you motivated and exercising so that you, too, can avoid a fall.

## What's My Dad's Take on the Exercises?

I asked my father if he'd be willing to comment on our exercise plan as part of this book. Here's what he had to say:

"I participate in my own rehab by actively following a regimen of exercises prescribed by my daughter, Amanda Sterczyk. This includes standing, sitting and lying down exercises. These exercises are repeated ONLY while they can be performed easily and stopped before pain sets in. The aim is to improve strength in joints used in standing, sitting and walking. These actions also improve my range of motion and balance. Overall, my recovery from a number of hospitalizations is positive and I remain optimistic about reaching an improved level of physical activity."

Two months after we first began down this road, I can tell you that my father is doing much better. He is more confident, stronger, standing more upright, and to me, appears happier. I hope that the exercises in this book and my first balance book, *Balance and Your Body*, will also help you stay healthy and happy — and upright! — in your golden years.

## Want to Hear the Best News?

Three months after I began working one-on-one with my father, he was getting ready to mark his 80th birthday. In our province, that requires a driving test recertification, which he passed with flying colours. He told me that the exercises we had been doing together helped him pass the test, and he's right. Even our provincial ministry of transportation agrees that strength and flexibility are just as important when you get behind the wheel.[1] It's not just about preventing falls when you're walking, it's being able to maintain your independence as you age. I still help my dad with exercises once or twice a week — both of our schedules make it difficult to consistently fit three focused workouts in a week. But my father feels more confident to

1. Ontario Ministry of Transportation, *Aging and Driving: Ontario's Licence Renewal Program for Drivers Age 80 and Above*, website accessed February 2, 2020, http://www.mto.gov.on.ca/english/driver/pdfs/ges-booklet-english.pdf.

continue exercising on his own on the days I can't be there. And he continues to increase his strength and improve his joint mobility—two key factors in preventing a fall.

## What's the Speed Limit?

When you move on to the exercise section, you'll see that many of my instructions say things like, "slowly," or "with control." My intention is to have you focus on controlled movement that helps to strengthen the muscles being targeted, but also to prevent a fall. You're doing these exercises because you've identified a need for improvement in muscle strength. Sometimes, we may want to rush moves—if, for example, we find them difficult and want to complete them faster.

But executing the sequences too quickly is problematic for a few reasons. First, you won't necessarily strengthen the muscles correctly because you will be relying instead on momentum to move, not muscle power. Second, you're more at risk from falling if you're rushing. One time, an older acquaintance told me she tripped and broke her wrist *because* she was rushing. You see, she didn't notice the slight lift on the curb as she rushed forward, caught her toe, and, well, you know how the story ends.

My father very wisely told me that he is more purposeful with his movements these days. He told me that he wants to focus on controlled movement and doesn't want to risk a fall. So he takes his time and pays attention to where he plants his foot. I hope you'll take the same care both with these exercises and with your day-to-day activities.

This also remind me of a book I bought years ago called *Self Defence for Seniors*.[2] In it, the author explains that self-defence changes as you age. No longer should you be thinking of a "fight your way out" scenario; rather, you should focus on getting out a scary situation safely and in one piece. The same goes for exercising. There's no need to be a hero. If you're reading this book, your fitness goals are about enjoying your golden years without injuries sustained from falls. So, here's my advice to you as you tackle the exercises:

- Take it slow,
- Take breaks as needed,
- Remember that Rome wasn't built in a day and neither were you, and
- Focus on the goal of your exercise plan (don't forget the training log in the appendix to help you track your progress—both the peaks and the steps).

And with that, it's time for us to move to the Action Plan, and get you exercising.

---

2. Ken Boire, Self Defence for Seniors: A Special Self Defence System for Seniors (Denver: Outskirts Press, 2014).

# PART THREE
# THE ACTION PLAN:
# HOW TO NOT FALL

*Mens sana in corpore sano.*
*(A sound mind in a sound body.)*
*- Juvenal, Roman poet (AD c. 60-c. 130)*

## Can We Review Setup?

These are exercises you can do in your home—with your doctor's permission, of course. As you start each exercise, focus on making slow, purposeful movements. If you feel dizzy, stop and sit down. If the feeling persists, consult your doctor.

Hang on to something solid if you need help with balance. If you're moving around, make sure the area is free of obstacles. Ask for help if you need it. If someone is watching you move, they can also help correct your position for optimal results. And don't forget that you're getting stronger each time you practice these exercises. Give yourself a pat on the back for taking ownership of your body!

If you read *Balance and Your Body: How Exercise Can Help You Avoid a Fall,* you may recall that I often exercise in my bare feet, but I know not everyone is comfortable in bare feet. Whatever you choose, the most important thing is that you're at ease when performing the exercises. For several of the standing sequences, you will see guidance recommending that you keep your shoes and socks on your feet, to prevent slipping.

The exercises are divided into three sections: standing, seated, and lying down exercises. If you're not comfortable getting on the floor for the lying exercises, you can do them on your bed. Each exercise is accompanied by one or two illustrations to get you started, as well as step-by-step instructions. At the bottom of the description, you'll find modifications on how to make an exercise easier or harder.

There are also two appendices to help you with the exercises. The first includes a chart with each exercise listed. It will help you track your progress with the exercises for the first two weeks, assuming you complete the exercises three times a week. The second appendix provides a breakdown of the exercises and what function they're targeting.

## Can We Talk Safety?

Before we proceed, let's talk about safety. As with other fitness texts, my book includes a disclaimer in the front: "The information in this book should not be used for diagnosis or treatment, or as a substitute for professional medical care. Before beginning any exercise program, consult your physician." That's not just legal jargon for the sake of it—it's important advice to heed because everyone's health is different.

But there's more: I want you to use your common sense. The tips in this book are meant to help you, not hurt you. If something bothers you, STOP doing it. The balance exercises are meant to improve your balance, not make you fall down. Always make sure you have something sturdy to hang onto—a counter, a wall, a chair that won't slip, or a fellow human, be it a relative, a friend, or a personal trainer.

If you have any questions at all about the exercises listed here, take this book to your doctor or other health professional and review it with them. Or you can hire a personal trainer in your neighbourhood to work with you. There are many great fitness professionals who work with older adults just like you.

And remember, the goal is to make you stronger and improve your balance. Even small increments of activity and exercise will get you closer to this goal. Shall we get started?

## Are You Breathing?

It's very important to remember to breathe as you complete the exercises. That's because holding your breath when you're exerting your body can place unnecessary strain on your heart. A helpful rule of thumb is to inhale and exhale for each step. For example: Inhale to complete step 1, exhale to complete step 2. Repeat. Depending on which part of an exercise sequence you find most difficult, you'll want to modify your breathing so that you're exhaling on the most strenuous portion. If you inhale during the most difficult part, you're more likely to hold your breath at the end of the inhalation.

## What About Warmups?

If you're wondering about warmups, let's chat about that now. The purpose of a warmup is to prepare your body for the exercises you are about to do, that is, the workout you're preparing to undertake. A warmup gets your blood pumping, gradually and safely increasing your heart rate and blood circulation. It loosens up stiff joints and delivers blood to the muscles you're about to use, preventing the risk of an injury.

Even if you're planning to tackle these exercises one at a time—i.e., one exercise per day—your body will still benefit from warming up for three to five minutes. But don't worry, it doesn't have to be complicated. Here are three simple moves you can do to get warmed up and ready to exercise:

- marching on the spot,
- shoulder rolls, and
- arm swings.

If none of these appeal, you can also simply turn on your favourite song and dance! You can also use music to keep time as you complete the warmup suggestions I listed above.

# STANDING EXERCISES

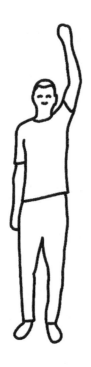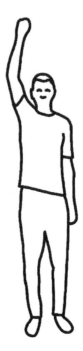

## Overhead Arm Raises

Our torso can help keep us upright for exercises like overhead arm reaches. This improves our posture, strengthening both our muscles and our bones. When we stand straighter, it is easier to walk with a straighter frame and see where we are going, thus reducing the likelihood of a momentum-based fall. These reaches will help you achieve that goal and keep you from toppling forward when you're walking.

**To start:** Stand tall with your feet facing forward, hip-width apart, with your arms hanging at your sides.

1. Lift your right arm above your head, straightening the elbow and maintaining a tall posture.

2. Lower your right arm to the starting position.

3. Lift your left arm above your head, straightening the elbow and maintaining a tall posture.

4. Lower your left arm to the starting position.

Continue alternating arm reaches until you have completed 10 on each side.

**Visualize:** You are a puppet, and the string holding up your head and torso is taut and unmoving, while the strings on your wrists alternately lift your arms upwards.

**Do you need to make it easier?** You can sit in a chair to complete the arm reaches.

**Are you ready to make it harder?** Try balancing on one foot to increase the difficulty of the arm reaches.

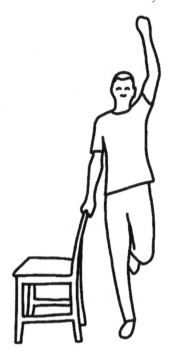

## Bird Dog

The bird dog exercise helps improve your posture by strengthening the muscles in your torso. It will increase your stability and coordination as you work on your balance.

**To start:** Stand beside a wall, counter, or sturdy chair. Hang on to your steady surface with your left hand.

1. Reach towards the ceiling with your right hand, making your arm as straight as possible above your head.

2. Lift the right leg off the ground. You can bend this leg at the knee to avoid leaning away from your support.

3. Hold this position—one arm up, one leg up—for as long as you can, up to 30 seconds. You may feel your body

swaying a bit as you balance on one leg. Maintain a firm grip on your support to remain stable. Lower your foot to the ground if you're feeling too unsteady.

4. Return to the starting position: Lower your right leg and right arm.

5. Turn around to face the opposite direction and hold your support with your right hand.

Follow steps 1 to 4 with your left arm and leg.

**Visualize:** Your arm is the nose of a pointer dog, and your body is a stiff board from your outstretched fingers, down your arm, across your torso, through your balancing leg into the foot on the ground.

Four modifications are listed below. The first two will make it easier, while the second two increase the challenge of the exercise.

**Do you need to make it easier?** Instead of reaching your arm above your head, lift it away from your body—to the side or in front—at shoulder height. Or, instead of lifting your foot completely off the ground, employ the "kickstand" position: turn your toes away from your body, slide that foot towards your opposite ankle as you lift it off the ground, keeping your big toe on the ground for stability. The sole of this foot rests against the inside of your opposite leg at ankle height.

**Are you ready to make it harder?** Try the balance exercise without holding on to your support. Or, take it to the floor: Begin on your hands and knees, stretching an opposite arm and leg away from your centre.

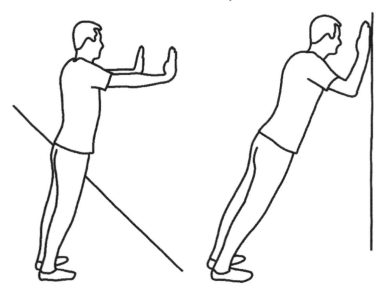

## Wall Pushup

Push-ups are an effective exercise to build upper body strength. Your chest, shoulders, back, and arms all work together to move you with control. Your abdominal muscles also play a role in maintaining a stiff torso and preventing you from arching your back, thereby strengthening your entire core.

**To start:** To avoid slipping, do this exercise in shoes or bare feet. Stand facing a blank wall or closed door, with your feet hip-width apart. Your distance from the surface will depend on the length of your arms, so you may need to shift your feet forward or back before you begin.

1. Place your open palms against the door/wall, directly in front of your shoulders. Relax your shoulders

down away from your ears, and squeeze your stomach muscles.

2. Check your elbows, they should be almost straight (not locked) in the starting position. Shift your feet forward or back until your elbows are at the proper angle.

3. Slowly bend your elbows to bring your nose closer to the wall or door.

4. Straighten your arms to return to the starting position.

Repeat steps 3 and 4 at least five to 10 times.

**Visualize:** Your body from your shoulders down to your ankles is a solid board, that moves as a single unit.

Four modifications are listed below: The first two will make it easier, while the second two increase the challenge of the exercise.

**Do you need to make it easier?** Walk your feet forward, and begin with a bigger bend in your elbow. If this is still too difficult, sit on a chair with your feet flat on the ground and your bum close to the edge of the chair. Follow steps 1 to 5 from a seated position.

**Are you ready to make it harder?** Walk your feet further away so that you're leaning at a sharper angle. Follow steps 1 to 5. For an added challenge, lift one foot off the ground. Perform five wall push-ups on one foot. Switch to the other foot and repeat.

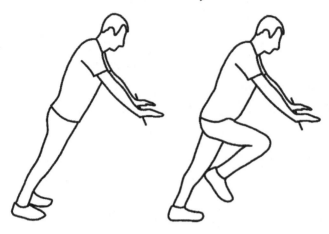

## Counter Knee Lifts

Also known as Mountain Climbers, counter knee lifts are a full-body exercise that work your legs, core, and upper body. They also qualify as a cardio exercise, as they help to elevate your heart rate. Performed against a sturdy counter, the angle will be less difficult than starting on the floor, which is described below as a modification to make the exercise more challenging.

**To start:** Place your hands on the edge of the counter, and walk your feet backward until your body is leaning at a 45-degree angle.

1. Pull your right knee to your chest as close as you can.

2. Lower your right foot back to the ground.

3. Pull your left knee to your chest, as close as you can.

4. Lower your left foot back to the ground.

Repeat steps 1 to 4 up to 10 times.

**Visualize:** Your body from your wrists, through your shoulders to your hips is a stiff, unmoving upside-down check mark. Keep your shoulders down and your stomach tense, moving only from your knees.

Four modifications are listed below: The first two will make it easier, while the second two increase the challenge of the exercise.

**Do you need to make it easier?** Bring your feet closer to the counter to decrease the lean of your body. Follow steps 1 to 4 in this position. If this angle is still too demanding, use a wall instead, placing your palms against the wall directly in front of your shoulders. Follow steps 1 to 4 in this position.

**Are you ready to make it harder?** Try to increase the speed at which you alternate pulling your knees to your chest. Want to make it even more challenging? Instead of leaning against a counter, complete this exercise on the floor. Begin in a plank position, holding yourself on your hands and toes. Line up your hands under your shoulders, with your legs extended behind you. Follow steps 1 to 4 in this position.

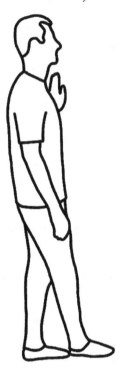

## Heel-Toe Walk

Heel-toe walking is a dynamic balance exercise that requires you to constantly shift your centre of gravity over a narrow base of support.

**To start:** Before you begin this exercise, make sure the surrounding area is clear of obstacles. Hallways are a great place to practice walking because the walls are close to you, in case you need to steady yourself, and hallways are typically clear spaces for moving about. If you are comfortable practicing outside, you can walk further. If you stay indoors, make sure you have enough space to walk at least 10 to 12 steps.

1. Position the heel of one foot just in front of the toes of your other foot. Your heel and toes should touch or almost touch.

2. Look straight ahead. Choose a spot ahead of you to focus on.

3. Take a step. Put your heel just in front of the toe of your other foot. Keep your gaze on your focus point to keep you steady and upright.

4. Take another step. Continue stepping, placing the heel of the front foot just in front of the toe of the other foot. Try to keep looking at your focus point.

Repeat for 10–12 steps.

**Visualize:** You are walking on a tightrope, suspended above the ground. Your feet need to stay in a narrow line to remain on the tightrope.

**Do you need to make it easier?** Start with your feet hip-width apart. Make your first step small so that you narrow the distance, but don't worry about trying to get your feet to touch (this may be too narrow for you to be comfortably upright). Stretch out your arms to the side, to increase your base of support. Or stand close to a wall and hang on as you walk forward, touching the wall without leaning against it.

**Are you ready to make it harder?** Keep going! Try to complete three to five minutes of heel-toe walking.

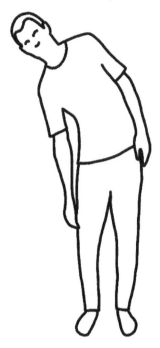

## Side Bends

Side bends work the muscles along the sides of your torso, helping to increase your upper body strength and maintain an upright posture.

**To start:** Stand tall with your feet facing forward, hip-width apart.

1. Place your arms at your sides, fingertips facing down towards the floor.

2. At your waist, lean to your right side with your fingertips reaching towards the floor.

3. Move back to your starting position.

4. Continue bending to the right and up again five to 10 times.

Follow steps 1 to 4 on the left side.

**Visualize:** You're a teapot wedged between two sheets of glass, tipping over from the waist without leaning forward or back.

**Do you need to make it easier?** You can sit in a chair to complete the side bends.

**Are you ready to make it harder?** Add a small can or light weight to the hand on your bending side.

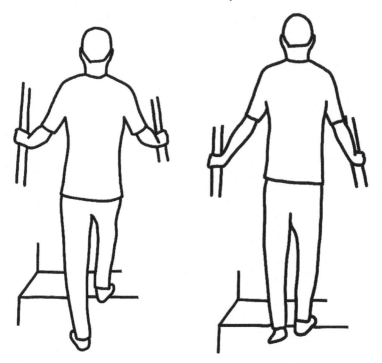

## Stair Step-up

Climbing a full flight of stairs can be daunting when your legs feel weak. You don't want to get halfway up and be stuck needing a rest, or worse, fall on the stairs. This exercise will help strengthen your leg muscles, boost your confidence, and improve your balance, thereby facilitating better movement when you have to lift your feet higher—like to climb stairs or to step over an obstacle.

**To start:** Stand at the bottom of a flight of stairs, facing the steps. Hang on to the wall and/or railing as needed for stability.

1. Lift your right foot off the ground and place it on the bottom step. This foot will remain here for the whole sequence, as this leg is doing all the work.

2. Straighten your right leg as you lift your left foot off the ground.

3. Place your left foot beside your right foot on the bottom step.

4. Reverse the movement: Lift your left foot off the step and return it to the starting position on the floor, bending your right knee as you lower your left foot.

5. Follow steps 1 to 4 for five to eight repetitions.

6. Return your right foot to the ground.

Repeat the entire sequence with your left foot remaining on the bottom step.

**Visualize:** A rocket in your foot on the step propels you to straighten your leg, thereby lifting the bottom foot off the floor with minimal effort.

**Do you need to make it easier?** Complete steps 1 to 4 once. Return your foot to the starting position, and repeat the modified sequence on the other side.

**Are you ready to make it harder?** Place your right foot on the second step. Complete the sequence at this higher height.

# SEATED EXERCISES

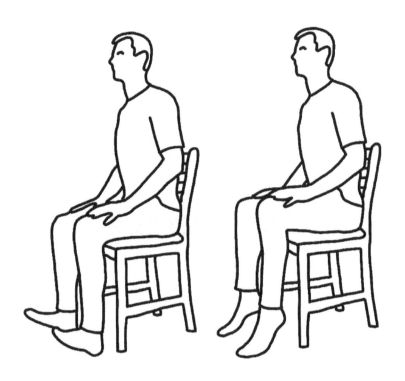

## Double Gas Pedal

The gas pedal sequence will loosen up stiff ankles and strengthen the muscles in your calves and shins, thereby making walking easier and more fluid. Sitting at the front of the chair, rather than relying on the chair back for support, will further strengthen your core (aka your abdominal muscles). This exercise can be done wearing shoes or with bare feet.

**To start:** Sit tall in a chair, with both feet planted flat on the floor, hip-width apart. Look straight ahead and keep your body tall throughout the sequence.

1. Moving both feet at the same time, lift your toes off the floor.

2. Lower the toes to the starting position.

3. Lift both heels off the floor.

4. Lower the heels to the starting position.

Repeat steps 1 to 4 at least eight to 10 times.

**Visualize:** Your feet are a seesaw, moving up and down in a controlled fashion.

**Do you need to make it easier?** Focus on one foot at a time, then switch to the other foot.

**Are you ready to make it harder?** Stand up to increase the balance difficulty of the movement. Hang on to the back of your chair for support, and follow steps 1 to 4 standing.

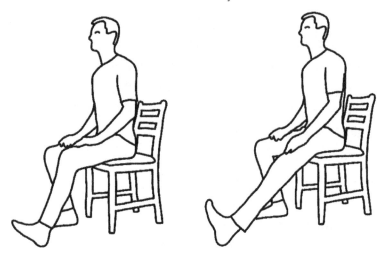

## Heel Slides

Heel slides work the muscles up the back of the leg, increasing lower limb strength and improving your walking stride. Sitting at the front of the chair, instead of relying on the chair back to hold your body upright, will further strengthen your core (aka your abdominal muscles). This exercise is best performed while wearing socks to allow your foot to move more freely.

**To start:** Sit tall in a chair, with both feet planted flat on the floor, hip-width apart. Look straight ahead and keep your body tall throughout the sequence.

1. Straighten your right leg and flex your right foot, so your heel remains in contact with the ground, but your toes are pointing up towards the ceiling.

2. Squeeze your bum muscles and the back of your thigh, using these muscle groups to drag your right heel

back towards the chair while it remains in contact with the floor.

3. Reverse the movement and slide your heel away from you, straightening your right knee until you reach the starting position.

4. Perform 10–12 repetitions on the right side.

Repeat steps 1 to 4 with the left foot.

**Visualize:** Imagine driving a car with no hand break and you are on a hill, slide the leg out to push down on the brake pedal (squeeze your bum muscles to hold it there). Then, release the brake slowly as you slide your heel back towards the chair.

**Do you need to make it easier?** Stay closer to the chair (don't straighten your leg completely).

**Are you ready to make it harder?** Slide both heels out and back at the same time.

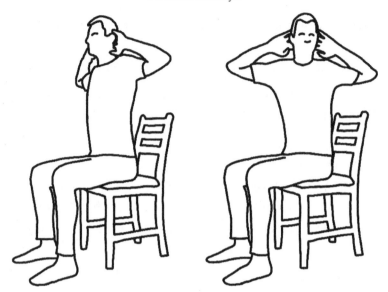

## Torso Twists

Torso twists work the abdominal muscles on the sides of your body, strengthening your core and improving the mobility of your spine. Both of these are important for maintaining good balance during functional activities, like twisting and turning as you empty your dishwasher or getting out of your car.

**To start:** Sit tall on a chair with your feet flat on the ground about hip-width apart. Make sure you don't lean back in the chair. Place your hands lightly behind your head, with your elbows bent and pointing out towards the sides of the room.

1. Slowly rotate your torso to the left as far as you comfortably can, keeping the rest of your body still, i.e. your bum doesn't move on the chair.

2. Rotate back to the starting position in the middle.

3. Continue rotating to the right side as far as you comfortably can, keeping the rest of your body still.

4. Rotate back to the starting position in the middle.

Repeat steps 1 to 4 at least eight to 10 times.

**Visualize:** Your body from your hips up to the top of your head is a key, turning as a solid unit back and forth in a lock.

**Do you need to make it easier?** Cross your arms in front of your chest to complete the sequence with a lower centre of gravity.

**Are you ready to make it harder?** Close your eyes to perform the torso twists, increasing the response of your vestibular and somatosensory systems.

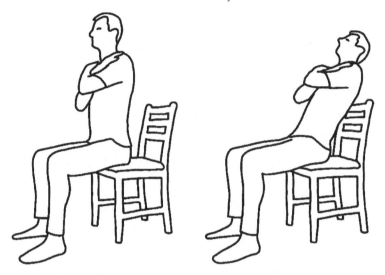

## Reverse Sit-ups

While everyone loves to hate sit-ups and other abdominal exercises, that's because they're targeting a part of our bodies that we often neglect. In addition to improving our core strength, sit-ups allow us to have better balance and stability, improved posture. They also reduce the risk of back pain and injury.

**To start:** Sit tall on the edge of a chair with both feet planted flat on the floor, hip-width apart. Look straight ahead and cross your arms over your chest, with each hand touching the opposite shoulder.

1. Slowly lean back, moving your torso as a solid unit towards the back of your chair. Stop before your shoulder blades touch the chair.

2. Pull your body forward in a smooth motion, returning yourself to the upright starting position.

Repeat steps 1 and 2 at least eight to 10 times.

**Visualize:** Tighten your stomach as if you're about to be tickled by your grandchild. Maintain that level of stiffness throughout the sequence.

**Do you need to make it easier?** Hook your hands on the sides of the chair, and follow steps 1 and 2.

**Are you ready to make it harder?** Bring your hands up beside your head, palms facing forward, elbows bent, with your fingertips touching your temples. Keep your hands in this position and follow steps 1 and 2.

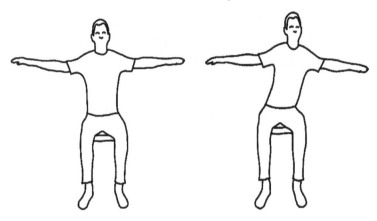

## Side-to-Side Arm Reaches

Side-to-side arm reaches work the abdominal muscles on the sides of your body, strengthening your core and improving the mobility of your spine.

**To start:** Sit tall on the edge of a chair, with both feet planted flat on the floor, hip-width apart. Look straight ahead. Lift your arms out to the side at shoulder height, with your elbows straightened.

1. Keeping your bum and hips planted on the chair, slowly lean your torso towards your left side, as if you're trying to touch something at shoulder height with your left hand. Don't tip your hand towards the floor.

2. Return to the centre, with your torso forming a straight line towards the ceiling.

3. Repeat the movement towards your right side.

4. Return to the centre starting position.

Follow steps 1 to 4 at least eight to 10 times.

**Visualize:** Your torso is bound by a metal cage, and your arms are the ropes in an evenly-matched tug of war.

**Do you need to make it easier?** Hook your hands on the sides of the chair, and follow steps 1 to 4.

**Are you ready to make it harder?** Follow steps 1 to 4, reaching even farther out to each side.

# LYING EXERCISES

If you're not comfortable getting on the floor,
you can perform all of these exercises on your bed.

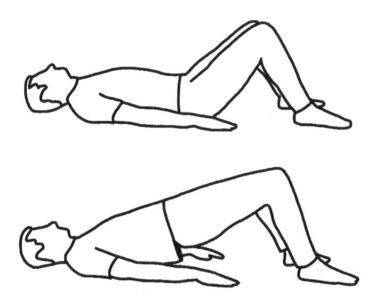

## Bum Lifts

Also known as a hip thrust or glute bridge, bum lifts will strengthen your gluteus muscles (that's your bum) and your hamstrings (the back of your thighs), which makes walking easier because these muscles help to propel your legs forward.

**To start:** Lie flat on your back, on your bed or on the floor, with your knees bent, feet flat, and your hands by your sides. Your feet should be shoulder-width apart. This is your starting position.

1. Pushing mainly with your heels, lift your hips off the bed/floor while keeping your back straight. Breathe out as you perform this part of the movement.

2. Hold at the top for one to two seconds.

3. Slowly lower your bum to the starting position as you breathe in.

Repeat eight to 10 times.

**Visualize:** Your hips and bum have a large band wrapped around them, that is being pulled upwards. This band makes your pelvis lift as one unit.

**Do you need to make it easier?** Don't push your hips as high into the air, only push halfway up.

**Are you ready to make it harder?** You can perform this exercise one leg at a time. Lift one foot off the bed or floor, follow steps 1 to 3. Lower that foot down, then lift the other foot and follow steps 1 to 3 on this side.

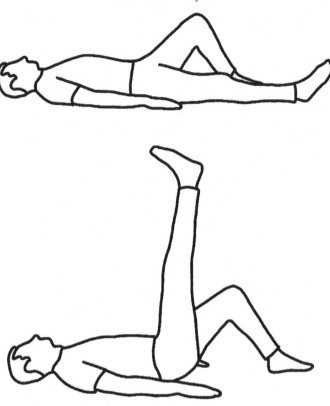

## Leg Lifts

This exercise strengthens the front of the hip, making walking smoother. It also helps to strengthen the core, as the abdominal muscles work hard to keep the motion controlled. Hint: Don't use gravity—lower your leg with control.

**To start:** Lie flat on your back, on your bed or on the floor. Bend your left leg at the knee and place your left foot on the bed or floor, to help protect your back during the exercise. Your right leg stays straight.

1. Raise the right leg as high as you can, keeping it straight throughout.

2. Lower the right leg slowly, with control. Don't arch your back as you lower your leg.

4. Repeat five to 10 lifts with your right leg.

5. Bend your right leg and place the right foot on the bed or floor.

6. Straighten the left leg.

Follow steps 1 to 4 with your left leg.

**Visualize:** A string tied around your big toe is pulling your leg towards your head. You are pushing a balloon towards the ground, directly under your heel. If you move too quickly, the balloon will float away.

**Do you need to make it easier?** Sit on the edge of a sturdy chair; straighten one leg in front and complete the leg lifts from a seated position.

**Are you ready to make it harder?** Place your hands under your bum, straighten both legs and lift them together. Don't arch your back as you lower your legs.

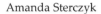

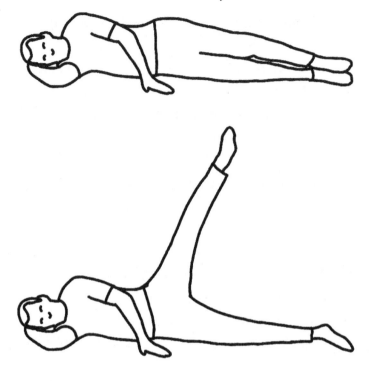

## Side-Lying Leg Lifts

A side-lying leg lift is beneficial because it strengthens all of your leg muscles and improves posture, flexibility, balance, and walking speed. It also improves range of motion in the hips, using muscles that aren't usually active in those who sit for prolonged periods each day.

**To start:** Lie on your bed or floor on your right side. Your body should be in a straight line with your legs extended and feet stacked on top of each other. You can place either your right arm or a pillow under your head. Place your left hand in front of you, palm flat on the surface, to keep you from rolling forwards or backward.

1. Slowly lift the left leg towards the ceiling, up to 45 degrees.

2. With control, lower the leg back towards your bottom leg.

3. Repeat for eight to 10 repetitions.

Roll on to your left side, and follow steps 1 to 3 on this side.

**Visualize:** You are lying between two walls that won't allow you to roll forward or backward. There is a string around your ankle that pulls your leg upwards. You are fighting the upward pull of this string as you lower your leg.

**Do you need to make it easier?** Bend your bottom leg before lifting the top leg. Avoid raising your leg too high throughout the exercise.

**Are you ready to make it harder?** Stand up to increase the balance difficulty of the movement. Hang on to the back of a chair for support, and follow steps 1 to 3 standing.

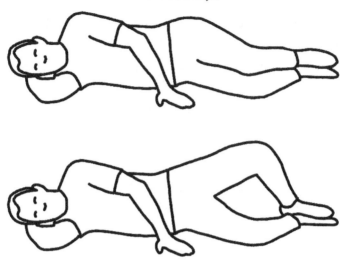

## Clam

The clam exercise strengthens the hip muscles on the outside of your legs, a muscle that is often neglected but is also beneficial in preventing falls.

**To start:** Begin by lying on your left side on your bed or on the ground. Support your head on your left arm or with a pillow. Bend your legs, pulling your knees in front of your torso, with your right leg directly on top of your left. Your heels, hips, and shoulders should form a straight line. This will be your starting position.

1. Keeping your feet together, lift your right knee upwards, directly above your left knee.

2. Pause at the top of the movement for one to two seconds.

4. Lower your knee to the starting position.

5. Repeat eight to 10 times.

6. Roll over to your right side, and repeat steps 1 to 5.

**Visualize:** Your knees are the centre of a clam shell that is opening and closing in the water. Your hips and feet are the edges of the shell, controlling how much the shell can open.

**Do you need to make it easier?** Don't lift your knee as high.

**Are you ready to make it harder?** Keeping your heels together, lift your feet off the bed or floor. Follow steps 1 to 5 with your feet in the air. Roll over and repeat steps 1 to 5 on the other side.

# APPENDIX A: TRAINING LOG

Below you will find a simple chart to help you track your progress with the exercises in this book. Across the top, you can enter the date or day you complete the exercises. Within the cells, enter the number of repetitions you completed.

| Exercise/Date | | | | | | |
|---|---|---|---|---|---|---|
| Overhead Arm Raises | | | | | | |
| Bird Dog | | | | | | |
| Wall Pushup | | | | | | |
| Counter Knee Lifts | | | | | | |
| Heel-Toe Walk | | | | | | |
| Side Bends | | | | | | |
| Stair Step-up | | | | | | |
| Double Gas Pedal | | | | | | |
| Heel Slides | | | | | | |
| Torso Twists | | | | | | |
| Reverse Sit-up | | | | | | |
| Side-to-Side Arm Reaches | | | | | | |
| Bum Lifts | | | | | | |
| Leg Lifts | | | | | | |
| Side Leg Lift | | | | | | |
| Clam | | | | | | |
| Notes | | | | | | |

# APPENDIX B:
# EXERCISE BREAKDOWN BY GOAL

The exercises in this book will help you strengthen your body, enhance your posture, and improve your balance—all of which will decrease the likelihood of a fall. The chart below highlights which exercises benefit which fall prevention goals. So, for example, if you only have a few minutes, and you want to work on lower body strength, you can easily see which exercises you might want to complete.

| Balance | Posture | Lower Body | Upper Body |
|---|---|---|---|
| Bird Dog | Overhead Arm Reaches | Bird Dog | Overhead Arm Reaches |
| Heel-Toe Walk | Side Bends | Counter Knee Lifts | Bird Dog |
| Stair Step-Up | Reverse Sit-Ups | Stair Step-Up | Wall Pushups |
| Reverse Sit-Ups | Side Leg Lifts | Double Gas Pedal | Counter Knee Lifts |
| Bum Lifts | Side-to-Side Reaches | Heel Slides | Heel Slides |
| Leg Lifts | | Bum Lifts | Reverse Sit-Ups |
| Side Leg Lifts | | Leg Lifts | Side-to-Side Reaches |
| | | Side Leg Lifts | Leg Lifts |
| | | Clam | |

# ACKNOWLEDGEMENTS

This book wouldn't be possible without my father's consent to share his exercise journey. To my parents, thank you for allowing me to help you age in place. I love you both. Many thanks to Suzanne Reid for writing a wonderful foreword. I really appreciate your help. Mélanie Fiala took time out of her busy life to share her expertise with me (and you). I value and respect your opinion, Mel. My friends Cassandra McCoy, Jeanne Wright, and Sheri Burge helped me fine tune the visualizations for the exercises. I really appreciate your help. Thank you.

As always, my editorial team—Kaarina Stiff, Dianna Little, and Matthew Bin—have elevated my work. I am so grateful for your expertise.

# REVIEWS AND TESTIMONIALS

"I really enjoyed *Balance and Your Body*! I had fun doing the exercises with my parents (aged 88 and 87). It gets them going, as well as me. It all makes sense—you have to read it and start exercising."

—Teresa

"*Balance and Your Body* is Amanda's second book especially written for seniors. The message is simple and true: "Move more, stay healthy longer!" The book is well organized and fun to read; the exercises are easy to follow and can be practiced whenever you have some time throughout the day (or sleepless night). No gym or equipment required!"

—An enthusiastic senior

"Her new book, *Balance and Your Body*, is very clear and easy to read. She explains why we need to move and the different aspects of balance. The exercises are simple and drawings help understand them. Not at all overwhelming to do the exercises. A very helpful book for any senior concerned about maintaining their independence. Essential for seniors to stay independent. Well done!"

—Amazon customer

"As a teacher and musician, I suffer from several repetitive strain injuries and back problems related to performance. *Move More, Your Life Depends On It* is a huge wake up call for so many of us who live our lives behind a computer and think there isn't any opportunity in our daily routine to exercise. Amanda's book showed me that there are countless opportunities throughout each day to exercise and reduce some of the chronic pain I experience just by doing my daily tasks. I highly recommend it for anyone in any industry."

—Danielle Allard, singer/songwriter

*"Move More, Your Life Depends On It* contains simple and powerful tips I have incorporated into my daily life. This book ranks as one of my favorites. The information is inspiring, timeless, well-organized, and an easy read. Amanda does a great job sharing her knowledge in a fun way."
—Fabiana Meredith, co-founder Qi

"Today while in four hours of meetings I got up and moved around...[I] even walked backwards to the door to excuse myself! Thank you for the tips...already making changes in my day!"
—Move More workshop participant

"Amanda, thank you so much for coming to talk to us at Retire-At-Home Services. Our jobs are demanding and require the utmost attention throughout our shifts. Many of our staff have continual neck and back pain due to the time they spend sitting & answering phones and typing. I really am thankful that you sent an important message to keep moving throughout our days. The simple tips and stretches you provided are invaluable to our staff! I believe every office would benefit from Amanda's presentation. Thanks again!"
—Catherine Bennett, Retire-At-Home

"I carry *Balance and Your Body* in my bag, between my cell phone and wallet, so I always have it nearby as reference. The exercises are basic and you can easily incorporate them in our daily life, and if you don't remember them, you can do what I do."
— Monique

# ABOUT THE AUTHOR

Amanda Sterczyk is an author and personal trainer based in Ottawa, Canada. In 2016, she founded The Move More Institute™, an initiative to promote healthy active living and teach individuals how to sneak "exercise" into their daily lives. Her slogan is "Move more, feel better." Amanda holds a Master's degree in social psychology from Carleton University. *Balance 2.0* is her fifth book.

You can connect with Amanda online by visiting her website: www.amandasterczyk.com.

Amanda Sterczyk

Balance 2.0

Amanda Sterczyk

Made in the USA
Monee, IL
12 March 2020

23060711R00056